Adaptations without delay

A guide to planning and delivering home adaptations differently

Endorsed by

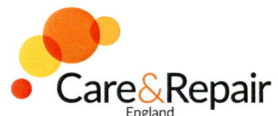

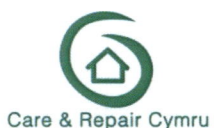

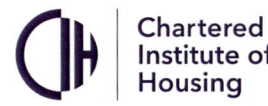

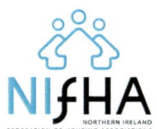

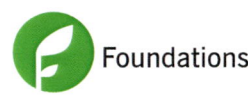

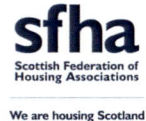

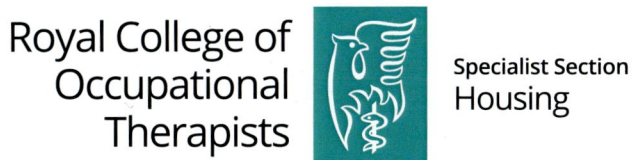

First published in 2019
by the Royal College of Occupational Therapists
106–114 Borough High Street
London SE1 1LB
www.rcot.co.uk

Author: Royal College of Occupational Therapists
Writers: Rachel Russell, Marney Walker, Ian Copeman, Jeremy Porteus

British Library Cataloguing in Publication Data
A catalogue record for this book is available from the British Library.

While every effort is made to ensure accuracy, the Royal College of Occupational Therapists shall not be liable for any loss or damage either directly or indirectly resulting from the use of this publication.

ISBN 978-1-905944-88-0

Typeset by Fish Books Ltd
Digitally printed on demand in Great Britain by The Lavenham Press, Suffolk

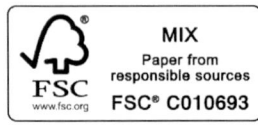

Contents

Executive summary

Introduction

The benefits of adapting the home are recognised as an effective way to improve the health and wellbeing of older people, and disabled adults and children. A more accessible home environment can improve independence, reduce risk and reduce reliance on assistance. As the body of evidence demonstrating the benefits of home adaptations grows, so does the recognition that the sooner they are installed, the greater will be the preventative benefits.

Across the UK there continue to be delays in the delivery of minor and major adaptations across all housing tenures. In recognition of this continuing issue, in 2017 the Royal College of Occupational Therapy (RCOT) commissioned the Housing Learning and Improvement Network (Housing LIN) to conduct a UK-wide review of *Minor adaptations without delay* (2006), which was focused on enabling housing associations to provide minor adaptations without the need for an occupational therapy assessment, and to identify whether a new version was required.

Review of current practice

The Housing LIN review was extensive. It involved a review of UK-wide policy and legislation related to the assessment and delivery of adaptations; stakeholder consultation across England, Northern Ireland, Scotland and Wales that involved telephone interviews with managers of occupational therapy services, housing providers, housing associations, home improvement agencies, and care and repair services; a nationwide survey completed by 800 front-line practitioners; and focus groups involving key personnel and organisations from the four UK nations.

The key findings of the review were as follows:

- A common theme in legislation and policy across the UK is the need for a more preventative approach to interventions, including adaptations, for older people, disabled children and adults, to maximise health and wellbeing.

- Waiting for a social care assessment is cited as a key factor in contributing to delays in the delivery of adaptations. Legislation pertaining to the funding of major adaptations has been misinterpreted as being dependent on an occupational therapy assessment.

- Current systems for delivering adaptations need to provide person-centred outcomes through a more integrated and collaborative approach to the assessment, design and installation of adaptations.

- In terms of demand for major adaptations, the most common are showers, stairlifts and ramps, often in situations that are simple and straightforward.

- Typically, the need for an adaptation has been defined by the *type* or *cost* of the solution, rather than the *complexity* of the situation.

- It is recognised that there is a large proportion of people who are not eligible for funding for adaptations who could benefit from better information, advice and guidance on how to get adaptations installed.

Adaptations without delay: a guide

From the review findings it was clear that a radically different approach to addressing the delays in the assessment and delivery of adaptations was required. This new approach sets out a better way of defining adaptations based on *complexity*. It focuses on the role of adaptations as a preventative intervention to support person-centred outcomes using an approach that makes the best use of the skills mix within the workforce.

The *Adaptations without delay* guide provides a fresh new approach. It has been developed in conjunction with those consulted during the review process and the RCOT's steering group. The overall aim of the guide is to reduce delays in the delivery of adaptations by providing tools that support a proportionate response. The guidance also ensures the valued and specialist skills of occupational therapists can be used to work with the growing number of individuals whose circumstances are complex.

The guide sets out the *Adaptations without delay* decision-making framework. The framework outlines the person-centred outcomes that can be achieved from having the home adapted. Workforce and operational factors to support integrated and new ways of working are identified. The framework outlines the different levels of *complexity* of the situation, rather than cost and type of adaptation. The levels of complexity are defined as:

- Universal (simple, low level).

- Targeted (straightforward, moderate).

- Specialist (complex, high risk).

The guide outlines circumstances when occupational therapists need to work closely with those with the technical expertise necessary to establish and develop bespoke adaptations and ensure that the installation is feasible. The guide highlights ways that occupational therapists can add value at a strategic level in the design of services, communication tools, and the provision of training and support for unregulated staff.

Practice examples from across the UK include:

- Training and support to enable support workers, trusted assessors and occupational therapy assistants to assess and make recommendations for major adaptations where the situation is simple and straightforward.

- Triage and duty systems at first point of contact used to identify whether or not the input of an occupational therapist is required to support a more proportionate and timely response.

- Integrated services that have established the right skills mix in the workforce in order to provide a proportionate response to reduce delays in the installation of adaptations.

- Services that recognise the value of occupational therapists' skills by focusing on complex cases.

The guide provides a list of what are considered to be the best examples of technical and design guidance to achieve the most accessible adaptations, as well as design to address the needs of people with sensory and cognitive impairments.

The guide is intended to have the following benefits:

- Ensuring a more responsive service to those needing adaptations.

- Reducing demand on occupational therapy services.

- Providing reasoning for key stakeholders about adaptations that do not need an assessment by an occupational therapist.

- Recognising the expertise of occupational therapists in complex situations where adaptations are required.

- Being applicable in all four UK nations.

Intended audience

The guide and the framework are intended to be used at a practitioner and strategic level by personnel in occupational therapy services, home improvement agencies, care and repair agencies, housing associations and other housing providers, but also by members of the public who need to know when to seek advice from an occupational therapist. It may also be of interest to health and social care commissioners and care practitioners where there is a need for an adaptation to help facilitate someone's care and support at home or reablement.

1 Introduction

There is widespread recognition that some simple changes to the home environment can completely transform the lives of older people, disabled people and children by enabling them to function more easily and safely in their own homes.

> The Equalities and Human Rights Commission found that approximately 1.8 million disabled people require suitable housing and approximately 300,000 do not have the adaptations they need in their existing homes.[1]

A growing body of evidence supports the view that home adaptations can prevent falls, reduce hospital admissions, reduce reliance on care, avoid the need to move into residential care and significantly improve quality of life and wellbeing for individuals, their families and carers.[2] At the same time, the retail market and independent builders are beginning to adapt to consumer-led changes. There is potential for a growing self-funder market across all tenures for equipment and adaptations.

A number of factors (including demographic changes) are therefore increasing demand for home adaptations. Yet across the UK there continue to be significant delays in the delivery of adaptations.[3] The UK Government's recent review of Disabled Facilities Grants (DFGs)[4] in England highlights that there is a pressing need for all services concerned to be able to provide a more timely response to installing adaptations that can deliver better outcomes for the person. In Wales, the Auditor General found that public bodies have a limited understanding of the longer-term benefits of housing adaptations, and there remains significant scope to reform the system to improve equality and wellbeing.[5]

---

1   Equality and Human Rights Commission (2018) *Housing and disabled people: Britain's hidden crisis.* [s. l.]: Equality and Human Rights Commission. Available at: *https://www.equalityhumanrights.com/sites/default/files/housing-and-disabled-people-britains-hidden-crisis-main-report_0.pdf* Accessed on 16.11.18.
2   Centre for Ageing Better (2017) *Room to improve: the role of home adaptations in improving later life.* [London]: Centre for Ageing Better. Available at: *https://www.ageing-better.org.uk/publications/room-improve-role-home-adaptations-improving-later-life* Accessed on 09.11.19.
3   Equality and Human Rights Commission (2018) *Housing and disabled people: Britain's hidden crisis.* [s. l.]: Equality and Human Rights Commission. Available at: *https://www.equalityhumanrights.com/sites/default/files/housing-and-disabled-people-britains-hidden-crisis-main-report_0.pdf* Accessed on 16.11.18.
4   Mackintosh S, Smith P, Garrett H, Davidson M, Morgan G, Russell R (2018) *Disabled Facilities Grant (DFG) and other adaptations reviews*: *external review*. Main report. Bristol: University of the West of England. Available at: *https://assets.publishing.service.gov.uk/government/uploads/system/uploads/attachment_data/file/762920/Independent_Review_of_the_Disabled_Facilities_Grant.pdf* Accessed on 12.03.19.
5   Auditor General for Wales (2018) *Housing adaptations.* Cardiff: Wales Audit Office. Available at: *http://www.audit.wales/system/files/publications/housing-adaptations-2018-english.pdf* Accessed on 12.03.19.

Whether based in housing, health or social care, occupational therapists have an established role in carrying out assessments and making recommendations for adaptations, partly driven by statutory obligations. Their specialist expertise is invaluable in contributing to finding the best solutions to support older and disabled people in their own homes. However, there is a significant proportion of situations that are simple and straightforward which may not require specialist occupational therapy assessment or interventions. This is particularly the case where the timely installation of an adaptation or a piece of equipment prevents or delays the development of more acute health and social care needs.

Purpose of this guide

HOW TO USE THIS GUIDE

This guide will enable you:

- **To reduce delays** by avoiding service design and delivery based on cost and type of adaptation.

- **To make more effective use** of occupational therapists by understanding the workforce skills and operational considerations required to deliver adaptations.

- **To reduce delays** where legislation and the role of occupational therapists has been misinterpreted.

- **To understand the type of situations** where an occupational therapist does not need to be involved in the assessment for an adaptation.

- **To develop or redesign service delivery models** based on person-centred and preventative outcomes.

- **To understand what level of home adaptation** service and help you might offer.

- **To ensure your organisation takes a safe and person-centred approach** to providing adaptations to older and disabled people.

The primary purpose of this guide is to address delays in the delivery of all types of adaptations (minor and major) across all tenures that occur when people receive a disproportionate response to their need for an adaptation. Delays in installing adaptations can increase the risk of health and social care needs developing or increasing. A person waiting for an occupational therapy assessment where the situation and need for an adaptation is relatively simple and straightforward should therefore be avoided.

The core principles underlying this guide are that the person is central to the process and that the preventative benefits of adaptations are maximised. The aim is to enable all services concerned with adaptations to provide a more proportionate and timely response, reducing delays in installation of adaptations and alleviating the likelihood of an unplanned hospital admission or an unwanted move to residential or nursing care. *The intention is that the widespread skills and knowledge of all professionals involved in the adaptation process are put to best effect.*

Intended audience

Adaptations without delay is intended to be used by practitioners and organisations across the UK who may be contacted by disabled and older people and their families who are seeking advice or support with home adaptations, including:

- Occupational therapists in health, social care and housing settings.

- Occupational therapists in independent practice.

- Housing association housing managers and officers, surveyors and property staff.

- Local authority housing managers and officers, surveyors and property staff.

- Care and repair agency technical staff and case workers.

- Handyperson services staff.

- Home improvement agency technical staff and case worker (England).

- Health and social care commissioners and practitioners in local authorities and the NHS.

- Members of Integrated Joint Boards (Scotland).

- Members of Regional Partnership Boards (Wales).

- Members of Health and Wellbeing Boards (England).

- Environmental health officers/grants officers.

- Voluntary organisations' housing staff/home visitors.

- Organisations delivering training on the assessment and delivery of adaptations.

- Individuals and their families who need to know about how to get adaptations installed.

The role of this guide for different audiences

Housing providers

Adaptations without delay builds on the previous publication *Minor adaptations without delay* (2006), which provided a rationale to support housing associations to provide minor adaptations without an occupational therapy assessment. Rather than providing a fixed range of minor adaptations, this guide will help housing providers consider how to provide a wider range of adaptations to their tenants without the direct involvement of an occupational therapist.

Local authority housing services, home improvement agencies and care and repair agencies

It provides a framework for considering the most appropriate response to a person's need for an adaptation. Based on the complexity of the situation, the framework will help those currently delivering adaptations to address the skills mix and operational considerations needed to deliver a wider range of adaptations without the direct involvement of an occupational therapist.

Occupational therapists

It provides tools to help occupational therapists articulate the value of their role in the adaptation process. By highlighting how their specialist skills and knowledge contribute to the adaptation process, the guide and framework helps to identify the circumstances when occupational therapists can be most effective in individual cases, at an operational level and in the strategic planning of services.

Health and social care commissioners and practitioners with responsibility for improving the delivery of adaptations

It highlights that delays in providing adaptations are often a result of the fragmented approach to the assessment, funding and installation of adaptations. Better integration of housing, health and social care provides an opportunity to consider how adaptations can be delivered without delay. It also sets out an overview of the *Adaptations without delay* framework (Section 3), providing those with strategic responsibility for integration or commissioning with an understanding of how the care and support of individuals with different needs can be addressed through different types of adaptation interventions to achieve improved person-centred outcomes.

Retailers, product suppliers and independent builders

Older and disabled people are becoming less reliant on, or are being signposted away from, statutory services. To adapt their home, many older and disabled people are directly purchasing products or employing builders. It is therefore vital that this sector provides safe and person-centred services. The framework can help guide retailers, product suppliers and independent contractors to understand when they need to consult with an occupational therapist for support to design and install the right solution.

Members of the public

While the guidance in this publication is focused towards those assessing and delivering adaptations, members of the public will also find the publication useful. A better understanding of how adaptations can help, and what kind of service they need to address the type of problem they might have, will help them to get an adaptation installed without delays.

2 Why *Adaptations without delay*?

DID YOU KNOW?

Preventing or reducing delays in people receiving adaptations can:

- Help people stay well at home for longer.
- Give people choice and control over their health and wellbeing.
- Help people have access to the wider community.
- Prevent or reduce the risk of falls.
- Reduce the need for formal care, informal care and residential care.
- Avoid unnecessary hospital admission.

In 2018, the Royal College of Occupational Therapy (RCOT) commissioned the Housing Learning and Improvement Network (Housing LIN) to conduct a review of the *Minor adaptations without delay* (2006) publication. This publication provided guidance to support housing associations to provide minor adaptations without the need to refer for an occupational therapy assessment. The review considered whether the guide needed to be updated, and if so, how it could be made applicable to stakeholders across the UK. The review method and findings are summarised in Annexe 2.

What the review found

The Housing LIN review found consistent policy themes and approaches across all four UK nations that are relevant to the provision of adaptations:

- Health and social care policy across all four nations supports a 'person-centred' or 'citizen-centred' approach. With regard to minor adaptations, this appears to support the policy of self-assessment and identification of own needs.

- Minor adaptations have a central role in the prevention 'agenda', including the reduction of falls, delaying admission to hospital, supporting re-ablement and recovery at home by enabling discharge from hospital or preventing a readmission.

- The process for delivering minor adaptations is done through a combination of integrated community equipment services, home improvement agencies/care and repair agencies, and by housing associations, with health, social care, housing professionals or older people referring into these services. However, in England, Scotland and Wales local authorities appear to take different approaches to how services for minor adaptations are accessed and provided.

- There is potential for better use of resources through a recognition that occupational therapists do not need to assess for adaptations that are required to resolve 'simple issues'. However, there appears to be relatively little guidance on defining the difference between simple issues and complex situations that need the expertise of an occupational therapist.

Across the UK, at both a strategic and practitioner level, the review found that:

- The greatest demand is for adaptations such as showers, stairlifts and ramps, which are often classed as major adaptations but can often be simple and straightforward.

- There continue to be delays for people who can self-direct their own care and wish to adapt their homes but are having to wait for a social care assessment from the occupational therapy service.

- There is a concern that delay in providing adaptations is potentially reducing the benefits of adaptations as a preventative intervention, for example impacting on their recovery or rehabilitation.

- With appropriate training and supervision, support workers, occupational therapy assistants and trusted assessors in many areas are carrying out assessments for shower adaptations, community equipment, assistive technology, stairlifts and ramps where the situation is simple and straightforward.

- In some areas the skills, knowledge and experience of occupational therapists are being used at a strategic level to develop policies, design guidance, triaging tools and training to ensure the right level of assessment and skills mix is used to make best use of local housing stock for existing/prospective residents, deliver tailored adaptations, improve the quality of the home environment and reduce delays.

What constrains providing adaptations without delay?

DID YOU KNOW?

The review found that barriers to delivering adaptations included:

1. Misinterpretation of legislation pertaining to the funding of adaptations.

2. A lack of research and evidence-based best practice guidance on the role of occupational therapists in the home adaptation process.

3. The assumption that if an adaptation is 'major' it is complex and must involve an occupational therapist.

At the strategic, operational and practitioner levels the review found that stakeholders want to address the delays in delivering adaptations, but they also identified barriers to change. The three main barriers were:

1. A misinterpretation of legislation (pertaining to eligibility for the funding of adaptations) has led to the assumption that a request for a major adaptation should be accompanied by an assessment and recommendation from an occupational therapist.

2. A lack of published guidance is preventing teams wanting to provide a wider range of adaptations, without the direct involvement of an occupational therapist, from developing the policies and procedures that would help with the risk management of this change.

3. Allowing the cost and type of adaptation to define the complexity of a case is preventing occupational therapists from concentrating their specialist skills on working with individuals whose circumstances are most complex and where they would have the greatest impact on the individual's health and wellbeing.

To reduce delays caused by the barriers identified by stakeholders, it was evident that a new type of guide was required in place of *Minor adaptations without delay*. Moving away from a prescribed list of adaptations and technical guidance, this guide introduces a framework to support the delivery of adaptations without delay.

This framework defines adaptations based on both the complexity of the situation and the type of structural alteration to the home. Based on person-centred outcomes, the framework identifies different levels of intervention, and what health and social care needs can be met by having the home adapted. There is also guidance on workforce and operational considerations required for the different levels of intervention.

3 *Adaptations without delay*: a framework for decision making

GETTING STARTED: What you need to know

- The framework describes three levels of home adaptations interventions: universal, targeted, specialist.

- There is a description of the person-centred outcomes expected at each level of intervention.

- The level (or type) of intervention is based on the person's care and support needs and the potential type of solution required.

- The framework includes three tables describing the nature of complexity at each level of intervention and identifies the workforce and operational requirements to deliver that level of intervention.

The design of the framework has been influenced by the widely recognised and influential Balanced System® of improving integrated care services for children[6] and the Comprehensive Model for Personalised Care.[7] Both these models link person-centred outcomes with the level of intervention that best addresses the health and care needs of the person. Using this approach ensures people receive a proportionate level of assessment and response to their needs while reducing unnecessary delays as well as demand for specialist practitioners and services.

To overcome the barrier that occupational therapists need to be involved in the assessment of *all* major adaptation because major adaptations have typically been defined as complex, the *Adaptations without delay* framework adopts a definition of adaptations[8] that considers the types of solutions alongside the complexity of the situation in four key areas:

1. The person, their priorities and needs.

2. The nature of the activities the person is having difficulty performing.

3. The environmental barriers to independence (physical, social etc.).

4. The types of solutions required.

---

6   See *https://www.thebalancedsystem.org*.
7   [NHS England] [2018] *Comprehensive personalised care model*. [London]: [NHS England.] Available at: *https://www.england.nhs.uk/wp-content/uploads/2019/02/comprehensive-model-of-personalised-care.pdf* Accessed on 12.03.19.
8   Ainsworth E, de Jonge D (2018) Minor modifications: it's not as simple as 'do it yourself' (DIY). In: E Ainsworth, D de Jonge, eds. *An occupational therapist's guide to home modification practice*. 2nd ed. Thorofare, NJ: Slack. 381–388.

This approach to defining adaptations recognises that a simple grab rail may be the solution to a complex situation. Conversely, a shower adaptation can be a solution to a simple problem. In the first scenario, the person benefits from the assessment skills of the occupational therapist who will consider a range of other factors that may impact on the safety and wellbeing of the individual and their situation. In the second scenario, the person benefits from the design and installation skills of a technical officer and builder.

The four types of adaptations are described in Table 1.

Table 1 Categories of adaptations (adapted from the framework for home modification service delivery[9])

Type of adaptation	Description
1. Simple situation requiring a simple adaptation or readily available off-the-shelf/retail solution.	Installation of this type of adaptation requires minimal disruption to the structure or fabric of the home and/or is a readily available off-the-shelf/retail solution.
2. Simple situation requiring a standard structural solution.	Installation of this type of adaptation impacts on one or two aspects of the home environment, involving structural changes but with minimal disruption. The adaptations may involve reconfiguration of the space, but this can be achieved through standard building alterations or installation techniques.
3. Complex situation requiring a non-structural solution.	A person has one or more complex key area of need (see above) which requires the non-structural solution to be customised for the person.
4. Complex situation requiring a specialised structural solution.	A person has one or more complex key area of need (see above) requiring a specialised structural solution. This type of adaptation requires substantial structural changes to the home environment. The solution will involve reconfiguration of the spatial layout and/or installation of specialist fixtures and fittings, such as height-adjustable baths.

9   Ainsworth E, de Jonge D (2018) Minor modifications: it's not as simple as 'do it yourself' (DIY). In: E Ainsworth, D de Jonge, eds. *An occupational therapist's guide to home modification practice*. 2nd ed. Thorofare, NJ: Slack. 381–388.

The *Adaptations without delay* framework: overview

Figure 1 provides an overview of the framework, illustrating the link between the complexity of the health and care need and the type of intervention that best addresses the person-centred outcome. The levels of intervention are divided into *universal, targeted* and *specialist* types of solution. A person's health and care needs are not fixed and will change over time; for this reason, it is important that this is considered each time a person approaches a service for support.

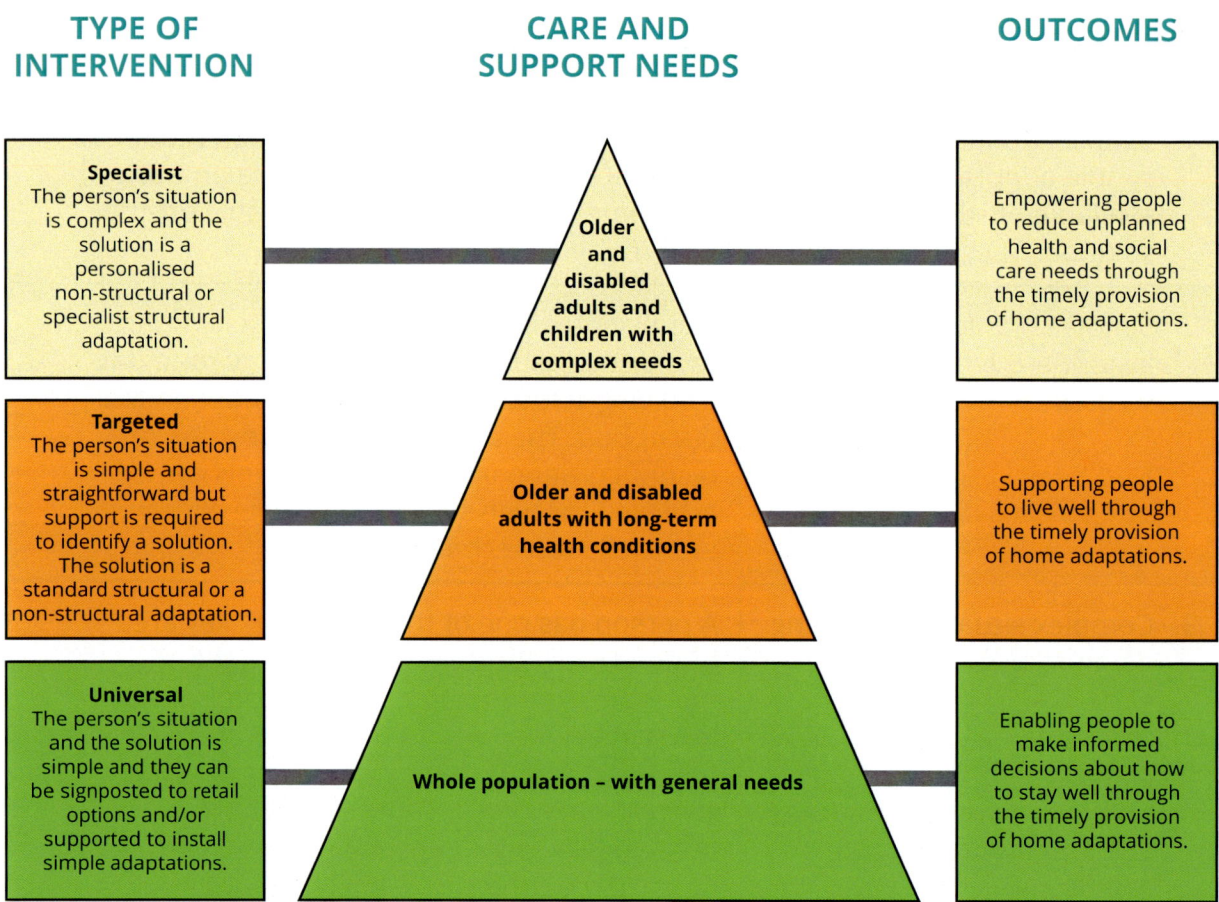

Figure 1 The *Adaptations without delay* framework

The purpose of the framework

The framework provides a holistic guide to the assessment and delivery of adaptations that supports positive risk taking for those who wish to explore different ways of working. It avoids disproportionate use of specialist occupational therapy services and offers a definition of adaptations that focuses on the outcomes for the person, rather than the funding mechanisms for the type of solution that is being installed.

The framework takes a person-centred approach that ensures the level of intervention is proportionate to the person's housing, health and social care needs. The framework:

- Outlines the circumstances when the needs and the solution are both simple and straightforward, and direct input by an occupational therapist may not be required.

- Provides a better understanding of the role of occupational therapists in the assessment, recommendation and design of adaptations, based on the complexity of the situation, rather than the type or cost of the adaptation.

- Outlines the appropriate level of workforce skills and governance required to meet demand and improve the delivery of an extended range of adaptations.

Using the framework to support decisions about the level of intervention required

This section explains how the framework detailed in the following tables can be used to understand the difference in complexity between *universal, targeted* and *specialist* types of intervention, the workforce skills and the operational and governance issues that need to be addressed at each level.

Universal types of intervention and services enable people with low levels of needs to make informed decisions about how to stay well through the timely provision of home adaptations. The solution is simple and they or their carer can be signposted to retail options and/or supported to install simple adaptations.

> Rita is struggling to get on and off her toilet. She contacts the local handyperson scheme to discuss her difficulties and arrangements are made to install a grab rail beside the toilet.

Targeted types of intervention and services enable older or disabled people with long-term health conditions to maintain their personal dignity, reduce risks and live well in their own homes through the timely provision of adaptations. The person's situation is simple and straightforward, but support is required to identify the most appropriate solution. The solution could be universal, but is likely to be a non-structural adaptation or standard structural solution.

> Robert was provided with bathing equipment several years ago, but he is struggling to use the equipment. He is visited at home by a member of a Home Improvement Agency. Through a discussion with Robert and an assessment of his difficulties, it is identified that the installation of a wet room will help him to remain independent with his personal care routine.

Specialist types of interventions and services empower people with complex health and social care needs to maintain their personal dignity, and reduce unplanned health and social service care needs through the timely provision of home adaptations. Due to the complexity of the situation it is likely the solution will be a personalised non-structural or specialist structural adaptation.

> Helen has multiple sclerosis and is finding a range of activities of daily living difficult to perform. Her abilities change from day to day. She wants advice on how to make changes to her home so that she can maintain her personal dignity, wellbeing and independence. An occupational therapist visits Helen at home. The occupational therapist works with Helen in the home environment and identifies the barriers in the home impacting on Helen. As part of understanding what type of adaptations Helen will require, the occupational therapist arranges for her to visit a demonstration centre. At the demonstration centre Helen is able to try different products and to look at options for adapting her home. Using the information from the assessment and visit to the demonstration centre, the occupational therapist visits Helen at home with a technical officer from the local authority housing team, who suggests several potential solutions. The occupational therapist works together with Helen to agree on the best long-term solution, and with this information an application for funding is made.

The following tables for each level of intervention provide detailed information about factors contributing to complexity at that level. Each table sets out the staff skills and operational factors that need to be considered to provide each level of intervention to achieve the best personal outcomes.

> ### KEY LEARNING: Benefits of using the *Adaptations without delay* framework
>
> The framework provides a structure for considering how current practice or future service design can be improved to deliver adaptations without delay by:
>
> - Providing a more proportionate response based on level of need and the complexity of the person's situation and type of solution required.
>
> - Establishing a workforce with the appropriate skills mix.
>
> - Acting as a guide to retailers and product manufacturers as to when members of the public may require a more targeted or specialist level of intervention.
>
> - Helping members of the public understand the level of intervention or type of service they need to adapt their home.

Table 2 *Adaptations without delay:* UNIVERSAL level of intervention

NATURE OF COMPLEXITY	WORKFORCE SKILLS	OPERATIONAL CONSIDERATIONS
Health condition is: • Predictable. • Stable. • No recent deterioration in health or wellbeing. **The need is related to:** • Reducing or preventing risk. • Enabling a person to maintain performance of basic activities of daily living. • Person and/or family can communicate and make decisions about their needs and the solution. **Complexity of the anticipated adaptations** • Person and/or family can communicate and make decisions about type of solution required. • The adaptation(s) being installed is an off-the-shelf solution and does not need specialising to meet the person's need. • It is anticipated the solution will be simple and intuitive to use and will not require any specialist training or support to use. • Person will require no or only minimal support to use the adaptation(s).	**Staff with:** • Knowledge and understanding of how health conditions and the ageing/developmental processes impact on the performance of simple everyday activities. • Knowledge and understanding of how to arrange the installation of a range of off-the-shelf adaptations that reduce / prevent risk or enable a person to perform basic activities of daily living. • Ability to signpost appropriately to local services including retail and handyperson services that can assist with installation of simple off-the-shelf adaptations. • An understanding of the circumstances when a person requires **targeted** or **specialist** input, including when it is appropriate to consult an occupational therapist.	**Accessing service** • First contact triage tool to identify if it is a targeted case. **Delivery of service** • Agreed policies, procedures and system for the delivery of adaptations provided without an occupational therapy assessment. • Agreed criteria for when to refer to targeted or specialist services or when to consult with an occupational therapist. • Agreed training and competency levels for non-occupational therapy staff who will facilitate process. • Agreed best practice guidance on the installation of off-the-shelf products. • Simple and transparent processes for procurement and installation of adaptations. • Partnership agreements between social care, health and housing agencies, housing associations, home improvement agencies and care and repair involved in the delivery of adaptations. • Effective review processes following installation of the adaptation.

Table 3 *Adaptations without delay:* TARGETED level of intervention

NATURE OF COMPLEXITY	WORKFORCE SKILLS	OPERATIONAL CONSIDERATIONS
Health condition is: • Predictable. • Stable. • No recent deterioration in health or wellbeing. **The need is related to:** • Reducing or prevent risk. • Enabling a person to maintain performance of basic activities of daily living. • Person and/or family can communicate and make decisions about their needs. • A visit is required to identify solution. **Complexity of the anticipated adaptations** • Person and/or family can communicate and make decisions about their needs. • The adaptation(s) being installed is simple and readily available, and if a structural solution (e.g. bathroom adaptation) it does not need specialising to meet the person's need. • It is anticipated the solution will be simple and intuitive to use and will not require any specialist training or support to use. • Person will require no or only minimal support to use the adaptation(s).	**Staff with:** • Ability to take a person-centred approach to identifying priorities, needs and preferences. • Knowledge and understanding of how health conditions and the ageing/developmental processes impact on the performance of simple everyday activities. • Knowledge and understanding of how to identify hazards and barriers to independence within the home environment. • Knowledge and understanding of how to identify and recommend a range of off-the-shelf and standard structural adaptations (e.g. stairlifts/shower adaptions) that reduce/prevent risk or enable a person to perform basic activities of daily living. • Ability to select and use appropriate documentation to procure adaptations appropriate to identified needs. • An understanding of when the complexity of the situation requires **specialist** input and when it is appropriate to consult an occupational therapist.	**Accessing service** • First contact triage tool to identify if it is a targeted case. **Delivery of service** • Agreed criteria for delegation. • Agreed policies, procedures and system for the assessment and delivery of adaptations provided without an occupational therapy assessment. • Agreed criteria for when to refer to specialist services or when to consult with an occupational therapist. • Agreed training and competency levels for non-occupational therapy staff who will conduct home visits. • Tools to support effective communication. • Agreed design standards and installation best practice for standard structural adaptations. • Agreed best practice guidance on the installation of off-the-shelf products. • Partnership agreements between social care, health and housing agencies, housing associations, home improvement agencies and care and repair involved in the delivery of adaptations. • Simple and transparent processes for procurement. • Effective review processes following installation of the adaptation.

Table 4 *Adaptations without delay:* SPECIALIST level of intervention

NATURE OF COMPLEXITY	WORKFORCE SKILLS	OPERATIONAL CONSIDERATIONS
Health condition is: • Unpredictable. • Changeable/fluctuating. • Including cognitive impairment. • Combined with physical/sensory/cognitive impairments. • Associated with being neuro-divergent. **Need is related to:** • Changing needs over time (child to adult). • Reducing or preventing risk. • A sudden change in health, independence and/or safety impacting on the identify and roles of the person and/or carer. • Safeguarding issues identified. • Advocacy needs during the assessment process. • Advocacy needs to make decisions about design of adaption. • Carers using adaptations as part of care package. **Complexity of the anticipated adaptations** • Several areas of home need adaptation. • The adaptation will need to accommodate the use of specialist equipment. • Installing adaptations could impact significantly on other members of the household. • Solution is non-structural or a specialised structural solution and requires both occupational therapy and technical involvement.	**Staff with:** • Ability to take a person-centred approach to identifying priorities, needs and preferences. • Knowledge and understanding of how health conditions and the ageing/developmental processes impact on the performance of simple everyday activities. • Knowledge and understanding of how to identify and recommend a range of off-the-shelf and standard structural adaptations (e.g. stairlifts/shower adaptions) that reduce /prevent risk or enable a person to perform basic activities of daily living. • Knowledge and understanding of how to select a range of interventions, including reablement, activity adaptation, energy conservation, moving and handling, advice and support for families and carers. • Ability to effectively communicate the details of bespoke adaptations and liaise with technical officers to find the best solutions appropriate to needs. • Knowledge and understanding of when an occupational therapy specialist assessment is not needed and it is appropriate to delegate assessment to targeted or universal input.	**Accessing service** • Effective triaging tool to identify complexity of situation. • Consider access to short-term solutions (i.e. equipment) while longer-term solutions are considered. **Delivery of service** • Person-centred process bringing together the assessment, design, procurement and installation of complex specialised structural solutions. • Integrated teams and/or joint working arrangements between occupational therapy and housing technical expertise. • Clear delegation of roles in relation to the adaptation process and who considers design requirements, writes technical specifications, designs technical solutions and supports procurement of the adaptation. • Effective and efficient procurement processes. • Effective review processes following installation of the adaptation.

4 How to use the *Adaptations without delay* framework in practice to improve delivery of adaptations

Introduction

Successful delivery of home adaptations is reliant on knowledge and understanding of what works best for the person and their situation. In practice, people need timely advice about what they might need, how they can get it and who can help them. This section considers how the *Adaptations without delay* framework can be used to achieve the above.

> **In this section you will learn how to use the framework:**
>
> - To provide a proportionate response.
>
> - To support the development of a workforce with appropriate knowledge and skills.
>
> - If you are builder, retailer or product manufacturer and want a guide as to when a person may require a more targeted or specialist level of intervention.
>
> - If you are a member of the public and want to understand the level of intervention or type of service you need to adapt your home.

How to use the framework to provide a proportionate response

> **Key message for achieving proportionate response**
>
> Getting the right response at the first point of contact, followed by signposting people to the right type of service (universal, targeted, specialist) reduces delays and the likelihood of people waiting on lists for assessments they do not require.

Signposting at first point of contact: At the first point of contact identifying and signposting people to the type of intervention/service they require reduces delays. The *nature of complexity columns* in the intervention tables (Tables 2–4, Section 3) can be used to support the development of tools to identify the type of intervention a person requires (based on the person's health condition, the nature of the need and the complexity of the anticipated adaptation).

Communicating the level of service delivery: Delays can be prevented when people are directed to a service that can best meet their needs. Services (including the retail sector) can use the *overview of the framework* and the *four categories of adaptations* (Section 3, Table 1) to benchmark the level of intervention/service they currently provide. This information can then be used to communicate what level of intervention a service is able to provide.

Supporting service development or redesign: Services can increase the range of adaptations they provide without an occupational therapy assessment if they address the workforce skills/knowledge and operational issues that arise when an occupational therapist is not directly involved in the process. The *workforce skills and operational considerations column* of each intervention table (Tables 2–4, Section 3) can act as audit questions to identify these gaps and issues, helping to support service development or redesign.

Strategic planning and oversight of adaptation services: A key recommendation from reports on the delivery of adaptations is the need to improve the strategic planning of services that deliver adaptations. The *overview of the framework* can be used to map and understand current assessment and delivery mechanisms in a locality. This information identifies gaps in provision, where improvement in pathways to access adaptations can be achieved and opportunities for integrated working or joining up of services.

Across the UK a range of cross-sector forums exist to enable continual improvement in the delivery of adaptations. In Wales this work is done by the Housing Adaptations Steering Group; in Northern Ireland by the Joint Adaptations Steering Group; across England the Home Adaptations Consortium champions quality of provision; in Scotland the Accessible Housing Group, which is a sub-group of the Scottish Government's Joint Housing Delivery Planning Group, involves a wide range of stakeholders and has a role in contributing to policy development, including on adaptations. The Scottish Housing Network is a membership organisation which runs a forum focusing on adaptations and mainly involves a number of local authorities and some Registered Social Landlords (the Scottish Government are invited to attend).

> ### Example: Strategic planning – establishing integrated housing support teams
>
> **Organisation:** The Lightbulb Project
>
> **Location:** Leicestershire
>
> **Services:** Housing support locality teams in each district council area. Targeted, proactive approach, including via GPs and other health/care professionals such as those in integrated locality teams.
>
> - Early assessment and triage of housing issues at key points of entry.
>
> - Hub-and-spoke model – integrated locality teams delivering minor and major adaptations, and housing-related support, advice and information.

Skills mix:

- Housing Support Co-ordinators (HSCs) and Technical Officer.

- Occupational therapists remain in Leicestershire County Council employment.

Method/process:

- Occupational therapists assess and recommend complex major adaptations and mentor/support HSCs (who are also trusted assessors) to complete less complex work.

- Housing specialists in a separate Hospital Enablement team identify housing-related barriers to discharge.

Impact and outcomes:

- Delivery costs, including Hospital Housing team approximately £1 million per annum against a potential £2 million per annum saving to health and social care reduced admissions/delays in transfers of care.

- Projected savings on DFG delivery costs through more efficient processes and staffing efficiencies.

Further information:

https://www.housinglin.org.uk/Topics/type/The-Lightbulb-Project-Switched-on-to-integration-in-Leicestershire

---

Example: Integrated service delivery

Organisation: Care & Repair Rapid Response Adaptations Service (RRAP)

Location: All Wales via 13 Care & Repair Agencies, Care & Repair Cymru and partners in statutory services – Health, Social Care and Housing.

Services:

- Very quick, responsive, small adaptations costing up to £350.

- Non-means-tested and available to all homeowners and private tenants aged 60+.

Skills mix:

- Care & Repair case workers, technical officers and handypersons.

- Hospital-based Care & Repair case workers.

Method/process:

- Referrals accepted from social care, housing, primary and secondary care health professionals, as well as direct requests from clients and their carers.

- Referrals can be community- or hospital-based, delivering quick solutions that prevent falls, reduce hospital admissions, assist independent living, or speed up safe transfers of care and patient flow within hospitals.

Impact and outcomes:

- Around 18,000 rapid response adaptations completed annually.

- Delivery times range from same day/immediate to eight days.

- Early engagement between hospital staff, patients and Care & Repair and consideration of housing needs at hospital discharge planning, combined with immediate practical solutions through RRAP programme improves patient flow at hospitals, and saves bed days.

- Care & Repair partnerships with occupational therapists, social care, health and housing provides quicker small adaptations in communities, outside DFG processes.

- Estimated that every £1 spent on RRAP saves £7.50 for the public purse.

How to use the framework to establish a workforce with the appropriate skills mix

Key message for establishing a workforce with the appropriate skills mix

The framework places older and disabled people at the centre of a process that ensures they receive the right level of assessment from a workforce that has the right level of skill and knowledge to assess and recommend adaptations.

Developing mechanisms for allocating cases: Delays are reduced when cases are allocated to the worker/practitioner who has the appropriate skills to manage the case to achieve the best person-centred outcome. For example, if a person's presenting situation is relatively straightforward, an occupational therapist does not need to be allocated a case where the anticipated adaptation is a standard structural solution, such as a bathroom adaptation or stairlift. The *workforce skills column* in the intervention tables (Tables 2–4, Section 3) can be used to support the development of mechanisms for allocating cases based on the *skills and knowledge* required to manage the case effectively.

Developing robust policies and procedures: Robust policies and procedures ensure workers/practitioners work within their scope of practice and are used appropriately to assess and deliver adaptations. This approach is particularly important when an occupational therapist is *not* involved in the assessment and recommendation of adaptations. The *operational considerations column* in the intervention tables (Tables 2–4, Section 3) indicates the policies and procedures that need to be developed and implemented at each level of intervention.

Example: Establishing agreed levels of responsibilities for making recommendations

Organisation: Royal Borough of Greenwich Occupational Therapy Service

Services: Occupational Therapy Service

Method/process: Guidance on scope of responsibility for Occupational Therapy Assistant Assessment Officers (OTA AO).

- Outlines criteria for when cases need to be referred back to an occupational therapist if they appear to become more complex.
- With regard to the RCOT code of ethics and professional conduct in relation to delegation.
- In line with agreed levels of professional competence outlined in the RCOT Career Development Framework.
- OTA AOs can assess and recommend simple level-access showers, stairlifts, half steps, hand rails, ramps, door widening, lever taps, window winders.

Factors where occupational therapy input and authorisation are required include:

- Safeguarding.
- Moving and handling.
- Clients with progressive, neurological and complex conditions.
- All children's cases.
- Complex social situations.
- Specialist and bespoke equipment needs.

Impact and outcomes:

- Reduces demand on occupational therapy assessments for major adaptations.
- Support for unregulated staff to assess and recommend adaptations when the situation is simple and to know when they need to seek specialist advice.

Developing and maintaining workforce skills and competencies: The *workforce skills column* in the intervention tables (Tables 2–4, Section 3) should be used to audit current staff for the appropriate level of skills and knowledge to assess and recommend adaptations for each level of intervention. If gaps in knowledge and skills are identified appropriate training can be provided. Where a service intends to extend the range of adaptations provided without an occupational therapy assessment then the workforce skills column will identify the skills and knowledge a worker will require to work safely and appropriately.

Example: Workforce training

Organisation: Housing Solutions Change Programme (Scotland) (developed by ihub Healthcare Improvement Scotland)

Services: Training a range of sector staff who may come into contact with people in their own homes, for example nurses, housing officers, podiatrists, occupational therapists and voluntary sector agencies.

Skills mix: Involves health, housing, social care and third-sector staff within local Health and Social Care Partnership areas across Scotland

Method/process: Training modules delivered by local training pairs (occupational therapist and a housing colleague) with an emphasis on early intervention, simple solutions, exploration of rehousing opportunities and personal outcomes. Partnership and an integrated approach are advocated to deliver better outcomes.

Module 1 promotes the value of 'early housing conversations' for any professionals visiting people at home to make use of opportunities for preventative interventions.

Module 2 provides a range of housing, health and social care staff with the skills to assess and commission straightforward adaptations where appropriate.

Module 3 trains non-social care occupational therapists to assess for and commission major adaptations.

Impact and outcomes:

- A wider range of staff are able to intervene earlier and enable forward planning.

- Enables a better use of skilled occupational therapists.

Developing interprofessional collaboration and practice for complex cases:

Delays occur when there is ineffective collaboration between occupational therapy and housing teams. Where occupational therapy and housing teams are not integrated, the framework and categories of adaptations can be used to support and encourage collaborative working practices. This approach is particularly important for complex cases where interprofessional collaboration and communication is essential during the assessment and design of the adaptations. Where integration of teams is being considered, the framework and tables are a starting point to consider the skills mix and operational issues that need to be addressed to provide a range of solutions to a population with diverse needs.

Getting the message across: effective communication

Effective communication between the staff carrying out assessments and the technical staff responsible for design and installation of adaptations is essential to ensure that completed adaptations are fit for purpose. It is important to provide staff with communication tools to make it as easy as possible to complete requests, make recommendations and explain the reasoning for key requirements.

In many areas around the UK standardised templates, which can be edited easily, are being used for simple straightforward adaptations. This ensures that good standards in relation to minimum space requirements, dimensions and key facilities are always included while being easily understood by technical staff.

Example: Adaptations Design Communication ToolKit

Organisation: Northern Ireland Housing Executive

Services:

- A published toolkit (including a list of adaptations that can be installed without an occupational therapy assessment).

- Evidence-based designs standards that can be used to help older and disabled people visualise the proposed adaptation.

- Standardised digital forms for applying for adaptations.

- Standardised digital formats for specifying adaptations.

Method/process:

- Published toolkit used to show older and disabled people designs of standardised adaptations.

- Electronic forms used to send information between occupational therapists and housing team.

Impact and outcomes:

- Improved older and disabled people's understanding of what adaptations will be installed.

- Improved interagency working and communication.

- Where standard solution can be installed, this has reduced need for joint visits.

Further information:

https://m.nihe.gov.uk/adaptations_design_communications_toolkit.pdf

How to use the framework if you are a builder, retailer or product manufacturer

Key message for builders, retailers and product manufacturers

Builders, retailers and product manufacturers are increasingly playing an important role in assessing, recommending and installing adaptations for people who are paying for their own adaptations. For the public to have confidence in this sector, it is important that builders, retailers and product manufacturers demonstrate they are implementing safe and person-centred practices.

Knowing when to consult with an occupational therapist: When assessing, recommending or installing adaptations it is important that builders, retailers and product manufacturers have the appropriate knowledge and skills to deliver this type of service to older and disabled people. The *overall framework and intervention tables* (Tables 2–4, Section 3) will help this sector to understand what level of intervention they can deliver safely and effectively, and when they need to draw on the expertise of occupational therapists.

Example: Supporting decisions on when to refer for occupational therapist assessment

A checklist used in Trusted Assessor Training

Method/process: An example of this is given in the Disabled Living Foundation training questionnaire:

How do I know when to refer on to an occupational therapist?

It can be difficult, especially when you first start working in the role of a Trusted Assessor, to know when you are able to provide a safe solution and when you are not. A simple way of deciding this is to ask the following questions:

- Does the customer have more than two conditions that are impacting on their ability to complete the chosen task?

- Does the customer's condition change significantly from day to day or is their condition likely to change significantly within the next year?

- Does the customer lack capacity to make decisions and/or are they unable to follow instructions?

- Is the environment complex and difficult to adapt?

- Is the solution outside standard and simple options available to you?

- Has the person lost the ability to transfer from one seat to another?

- Does a Trusted Assessor solution impact others' health, development or independence within the environment?

- Are there other areas that the customer is struggling with in the same environment that a Trusted Assessor solution wouldn't solve safely?

If the answer is yes to any of these questions then you should seek help from an occupational therapist.

Further information:

https://www.dlf.org.uk

Collaborative opportunities with independent occupational therapists: There are a growing number of older and disabled people who require a targeted or specialist level of intervention/service but who are self-funding. There is an opportunity for independent occupational therapists and building professionals to collaborate to meet this demand. The *overall framework, intervention tables and categories of adaptations* (Tables 2–4, Section 3) can provide a foundation and structure to develop business partnerships between independent occupational therapists and builders interested in providing a service to this population of older and disabled people.

Product suppliers and manufacturers' role in the delivery of specialist interventions: Sourcing, researching and analysing the cost–benefits of products comprise an important part of assessing and recommending adaptations. This process can be lengthy if workers/practitioners do not have easy access to product information. Product manufacturers and suppliers can play an important role in reducing delays in the adaptations process by making the following information available:

- How the product can be used to improve functional performance.
- What issues the product can/cannot address.
- Cost–benefit analysis of a product.
- Case study examples of how the product has been used in the real world.

How to use the framework if you are a member of the public

Key message to members of the public who want to use the framework to understand the level of intervention or type of service they need to adapt their home

The framework and supporting tables help you to understand the type of advice or support you or your family member need to adapt the home. Understanding this information will help you to make informed decisions about which services can provide the best solutions for your situation.

Identifying the type of intervention/service you or a family member need to adapt the home: Delays are avoided when people know the type of adaptation or service that will provide them or their family member with the best outcome to address the issues they are having in and around the home. The *nature of complexity columns* in the intervention tables (Tables 2–4, Section 3) can be used by people to understand the type of service and category of adaptation they are likely to require for each level of intervention. As discussed under *signposting at first point of contact* (above), communicating this information helps direct people to the service that best addresses their needs.

Example: Guided advice and support on daily living for older and disabled people and children

AskSARA is an online interactive self-help tool that guides users through a number of simple questions about their abilities and environment, and provides impartial advice and information on products and equipment to suit their needs.

Further information:

https://asksara.dlf.org.uk

Self-funding and checking the quality of a service: If you are self-funding an adaptation, it is important to know that the builder or company has the right skills to be able to recommend and install the adaptation. It is also important to know whether you will benefit from the input of an occupational therapist, who can assess the person and the home environment and then identify and recommend solutions. The workforce skills column for each level of intervention can be used as a checklist to ensure a builder has the right skills and knowledge to recommend and install the adaptation; in addition it will indicate whether you will require input from an occupational therapist.

Example: One-stop shop enabling self-referral across tenure

Organisation: Borders Care and Repair commissioned by Eildon Housing in partnership with Scottish Borders Council Housing Strategy

Services:

- Help and advice on housing repairs, improvements and adaptations.

- Scope: older people and people with disabilities living in the Scottish Borders, who are owner occupiers or living in privately or socially rented accommodation.

Method/process:

- One-stop shop for adaptations.

- Options appraisal templates to support decisions.

- Occupational therapy input on complex and high-cost cases.

Impact and outcomes:

- A consistent and equitable adaptation service to all people in the Borders regardless of tenure.

- Enabling people to self-refer for assessment and adaptations.

- Reduced waiting times.

Further information:

https://www.scotborders.gov.uk/info/20070/care_at_home/520/care_and_repair_service

Sources of design guidance

This section provides links to a range of useful sources of guidance, tools and relevant resources that can be used when considering the design of inclusive and accessible home adaptations. It includes links to guidance about factors to consider in designing for:

- Adaptations.

- Inclusive and accessible housing.

- Cognitive impairments.

- Visual impairments.

It is important when making recommendations for adaptations that practitioners are aware of their respective responsibilities in relation to *The Construction (Design and Management) Regulations 2015* (CDM 2015).[10] Services are advised to consult these when developing any operational guidance for their staff.

Adaptations

The aim of home adaptations is to make it easier and safer for people to access and use their own homes. There will be specific factors to consider for each individual, their priorities and needs, and aspects particular to their home environment. The following evidence-based guidance on space requirements and layouts provides useful baselines from which to develop bespoke adaptations.

Northern Ireland Housing Executive

Adaptations design communications toolkit is published by Northern Ireland Housing Executive and developed through close work and interagency working with disabled people, occupational therapists, housing designers and the Northern Ireland Federation of Housing Associations.

This toolkit provides detailed recommendations on space requirements and positioning to support the design of bespoke home adaptations. A useful tool to appraise room layouts, it provides evidence-based, consistent and equitable housing adaptation design standards for all housing tenures:

- Design formats that help visualise proposed housing adaptations and depict how people with mobility difficulties and carers use the space are included.

---

10 Health and Safety Executive (2015) *Managing health and safety in construction: Construction (Design and Management) Regulations 2015.* [London]: Stationery Office. Available at: *http://www.hse.gov.uk/pUbns/priced/l153.pdf* Accessed on 12.03.19.

- Standardised and robust occupational therapy formats for housing adaptations recommendations, financial governance, specifications and follow-up communications to all housing providers.

https://www.housinglin.org.uk/_assets/Resources/Housing/OtherOrganisation/adaptations_design_communications_toolkit.pdf

Muscular Dystrophy UK

Adaptations manual: for children and adults with muscle wasting conditions, revised for Muscular Dystrophy UK by occupational therapists who work closely with families living with muscle-wasting conditions, includes examples and practical information about what is available to families, as well as an outline of the process of making adaptations to their homes.

https://www.musculardystrophyuk.org/about-muscle-wasting-conditions/information-factsheets/equipment-and-adaptations/adaptations-manual/

Disabled Living Foundation

The Disabled Living Foundation produces a number of factsheets for the public, written and peer-reviewed by experienced occupational therapists, on factors to consider when selecting daily living equipment and adaptations. These include:

- Choosing and fitting grab rails.
- Choosing equipment for getting up and down stairs.

https://www.dlf.org.uk/content/factsheets-groups

Foundations

The national body for home improvement agencies in England provides useful guidance on the factors to consider when designing different types of home adaptations including:

- Ramp design.
- Shower adaptations.
- Kitchen adaptations.

https://www.foundations.uk.com

Care and Repair England

This national charitable organisation, set up to improve the homes and living conditions of older people, offers a range of useful resources on repairs and adaptations.

http://careandrepair-england.org.uk

Care and Repair Cymru

The national body for care and repair in Wales, whose vision is a Wales where all older people can live independently in warm, safe and accessible homes.

https://www.careandrepair.org.uk

Care and Repair Scotland

This body offers independent advice and assistance to help older and disabled homeowners repair, improve or adapt their homes.

http://www.careandrepairscotland.co.uk

Design Council

The Design Council's purpose is to make life better by design. They are an independent charity whose vision is a world where the role and value of design is recognised as a fundamental value, enabling happier, healthier and safer lives for all. Their current Spark programme is focused on home innovation and looking to turn bright ideas into products that transform the experience of getting around, remembering things and doing daily tasks to enable more independent living.

https://www.designcouncil.org.uk/what-we-do/accelerator/design-council-spark

Dunhill Medical Trust

The Dunhill Medical Trust not only funds the very best of the UK's academic and clinical research into understanding the mechanisms of ageing and treating age-related diseases and frailty, they also support community-based organisations that are working to enhance the lives of those who need extra support in later life. They have recently announced a new research programme that will address the evidence gap on adaptations and assistive technology to enable safer, independent living with dignity.

https://dunhillmedical.org.uk/2018/09/03/expert-in-the-future-of-housing-for-an-ageing-population-take-a-look-at-our-latest-call-for-proposals/

Inclusive and accessible housing

There are a number of resources available to support the design, build and retrofitting of inclusive and accessible housing. The core intention is to create homes that are flexible and adaptable to meet a range of needs.

Housing Learning and Improvement Network

The Housing Learning and Improvement Network (Housing LIN) brings together housing, health and social care professionals in England, Wales and Scotland to exemplify innovative housing solutions for an ageing population.

Occupational therapists: helping to get the housing design right is a collection of links to resources to support inclusive and accessible housing design.

https://www.housinglin.org.uk/Topics/browse/Design-building/occupational-therapy

An occupational therapist's access checklist: a practical tool is a quick reference checklist to existing regulations and best practice guidance on inclusive and accessible housing design, covering minimum requirements to more generous provision. Key aspects of the home are included, from access and approach to internal layouts.

https://www.housinglin.org.uk/Topics/type/An-Occupational-Therapists-Access-Checklist-a-practical-Tool

Royal Institute of British Architects

The Royal Institute of British Architects is a global professional membership body driving excellence in architecture. It supports its members to deliver better buildings and places, stronger communities and a sustainable environment.

The third edition of the *Wheelchair housing design guide* (2018) provides advice and design considerations to support the delivery of good-quality wheelchair-accessible housing. It details how to meet and exceed the minimum requirements laid out in *The building regulations: approved document M: volume 1: dwellings: category 3: wheelchair accessible* (ADM4(3)).[11] It was produced by contributors from the Royal Institute of British Architects, Centre for Accessible Environments and the Royal College of Occupational Therapists Specialist Section – Housing, along with input from a cross-section of experts including building control, architects, developers and other housing professionals. It includes:

- Clear cross-references to ADM4(3).

- Technical diagrams illustrating design details.

- Simple-to-follow guidance on best practice and technical provisions.

https://www.habinteg.org.uk/whdg3

Age-friendly housing: future design for older people (Park and Porteus 2018) sets out how we should approach the design of future housing for an ageing population. It looks at how well-designed, accessible and adaptable buildings can facilitate the provision of care, support, independence and wellbeing, and also includes a section on adaptation and refurbishment.

https://www.ribabookshops.com/item/age-friendly-housing-future-design-for-older-people/91915

---

11 Great Britain. HM Government (2015) *The building regulations: approved document M: access to and use of buildings: volume 1: dwellings*. [Newcastle Upon Tyne]: NBS. Available at: *https://assets.publishing.service.gov.uk/government/uploads/system/uploads/attachment_data/file/540330/BR_PDF_AD_M1_2015_with_2016_amendments_V3.pdf* Accessed on 13.03.19.

Royal College of Occupational Therapists Specialist Section – Housing (RCOTSS-H)

RCOTSS-H provides a forum for occupational therapists with an interest in housing, inclusive design and accessible home environments. It works closely with other organisations and professionals to advocate for improved standards of housing for older and disabled people.

https://www.rcot.co.uk/about-us/specialist-sections/housing-rcot-ss

Centre for Ageing Better

The Centre for Ageing Better is a charity, funded by an endowment from the National Lottery Community Fund, working to create a society where everyone enjoys a good later life. Their Safe and Accessible Homes programme of work seeks to ensure new homes are future-proofed and that there is a diversity of suitable homes, that current homes are adapted, and better information is available for people approaching later life.

https://www.ageing-better.org.uk/our-work/safe-accessible-homes

Centre for Accessible Environments

The Centre for Accessible Environments is a leading authority on inclusive design. It provides consultancy, training and research. It also has a selection of free publications and others for sale on building design and management to meet all user needs, including disabled and older people.

https://cae.org.uk/

Cognitive impairments

The design of the environment can have a significant impact on the abilities of people with cognitive and neuro-diverse impairments to make sense of their surroundings and support independence. This may include people living with dementia, learning disability or autistic spectrum disorders. The following provide some guidance on the factors to consider.

Beyond Accessibility

Beyond Accessibility is a team of therapists that specialises in how people live in the home environment.

99 ideas to make homes easier, safer, and more enjoyable for families with children on the autism spectrum by Paige Hays (2017) provides ideas and recommendations specific to designing home areas for families with members who have ASD.

http://beyondaccessibility.com/homes-autism-spectrum-disorder

The Challenging Behaviour Foundation

The Challenging Behaviour Foundation (CBF) is a charity for people with severe learning disabilities who display behaviour described as challenging. CBF provides information and resources to enable families to work with others to plan proactively for personalised housing for their relative.

https://www.challengingbehaviour.org.uk

Helen Hamlyn

The Helen Hamlyn Centre for Design at the Royal College of Art undertakes design research and projects with industry that will contribute to improving people's lives.

Living in the community: housing design for adults with autism (Brand 2010) details the findings from a research partnership between the Kingswood Trust and Helen Hamlyn, with a particular focus on housing providers, architects and designers involved in the design, refurbishment and development of residential accommodation for adults with autism.

https://www.rca.ac.uk/documents/390/Living_in_the_Community.pdf

Centre for Excellence in Universal Design: National Disability Authority

The Centre for Excellence in Universal Design is dedicated to enabling the design of environments that can be accessed, understood and used regardless of age, size and ability.

Universal Design guidelines: dementia friendly dwellings for people with dementia, their families and carers was published in 2015 by the National Disability Authority in Northern Ireland to inform those who commission, design, build, provide and occupy dwellings. The Universal Design dementia-friendly approach aims to help people to remain living at home and in their community independently and safely for as long as possible.

http://universaldesign.ie

Dementia Services Development Centre (DSDC), University of Stirling

The DSDC is an international centre of knowledge and expertise dedicated to improving the lives of people with dementia. It draws on research and practice from across the world to provide a comprehensive, up-to-date resource on all aspects of dementia.

https://dementia.stir.ac.uk/about-dsdc

Visual impairment

Attention to levels and location of lighting and tonal contrast can have a significant impact on the ability of people with sight loss to find their way around, and help to make it easier and safer to carry out everyday activities.

Housing Learning and Improvement Network

A comprehensive range of information on design and lighting for people with sight loss is available on dedicated pages.

https://www.housinglin.org.uk/Topics/browse/sight-loss-home-the-built-environment/

Thomas Pocklington Trust

Thomas Pocklington Trust is a national charity dedicated to delivering positive change for people with sight loss. The Trust funds research to support independent living and identify barriers and opportunities in areas such as employment, housing and technology.

Making an entrance: colour, contrast and design of entrances to homes of people with sight loss (2013)

http://pocklington-trust.org.uk/wp-content/uploads/2016/02/Check-List.pdf

Lighting in and around the home: a guide to better lighting for people with sight loss (2018)

http://www.pocklington-trust.org.uk/project/lighting-around-home-guide-better-lighting-people-sight-loss

Good practice in the design of homes and living spaces for people with dementia and sight loss (Greasley-Adams et al. 2011; jointly produced by Thomas Pocklington Trust and DSDC)

http://dementia.stir.ac.uk/design/good-practice-design-dementia-and-sight-loss

Royal National Institute of Blind People

RNIB is one of the UK's leading sight loss charities and the largest community of blind and partially sighted people. They have a dedicated webpage that provides useful information for people who are losing their sight or have a sight problem. It explains the types of improvements, repairs or adaptations that may be needed to help people with sight loss live independently.

https://www.rnib.org.uk/information-everyday-living-home-and-leisure/adapting-your-home

Annexe 2
Review method and findings

The Royal College of Occupational Therapists (RCOT) commissioned a team from the Housing Learning and Improvement Network (Housing LIN), which included occupational therapists, to:

- Determine whether there was still a need for *Minor adaptations without delay* publication, Part 1.

- Determine whether there was still a need for *Minor adaptations without delay* publication, Part 2 (Technical Specifications).

- Ensure that a revised version of *Minor adaptations without delay* was produced that would be valued by key stakeholders in all four UK nations and representative of occupational therapy practice.

- Raise the profile of the assessment process of occupational therapists in preventative adaptations and demonstrate when their expertise is required.

The original version of *Minor adaptations without delay* (MAWD), which was published in 2006, was jointly commissioned by the College of Occupational Therapists and the former Housing Corporation. The guidance was in two parts:

- Part 1: A practical guide for housing associations, which included a list of minor adaptations that do not require an occupational therapy assessment and outlined the criteria for good practice in the delivery.

- Part 2: Technical Specifications, which provided guidance on the installation of a selection of minor adaptations.

The primary aim of MAWD was to enable more timely delivery of minor adaptations for tenants of housing associations.

The review of MAWD, undertaken during 2018, involved:

- A desktop review of current policy, legislation, guidance and key research of relevance to the delivery and benefits of home adaptations across the four UK nations.

- Primary research, which involved:
  - Interviews with 31 professional stakeholders (January to April 2018).
  - An online survey aimed at front-line practitioners that generated over 800 responses.
  - Discussion groups with stakeholders in all four UK nations (May/June 2018).

Interviews were conducted with:

- Occupational therapy managers.
- Occupational therapy policy leads in the four UK nations.
- Housing associations.
- National bodies for home improvement agencies.
- Care and repair organisations.
- Royal College of Occupational Therapists Specialist Section – Housing leads in the four UK nations.

Focus group meetings were subsequently held in all four UK nations, which included groups in Scotland, Northern Ireland and Wales, a practitioner consultation meeting in Manchester, and a presentation at the Home Adaptations Consortium, England. The consultation also included a joint meeting as part of the Disabled Facilities Grant Review in England.

The purpose of this primary research was to:

- Assess the extent to which the original MAWD publication achieved its aims.
- Across the four nations, identify the common issues affecting the process of providing (minor) adaptations.
- Elicit the gaps stakeholders identified in the original publication.
- Identify the content and resources required in a new *Adaptations without delay* guide.

Findings in relation to the extent to which MAWD has achieved its aims included:

- For the housing associations MAWD was targeted at, it has been and continues to be a valuable resource (but some housing associations are unaware of MAWD).
- Occupational therapy managers have used it as a negotiation tool with housing associations in relation to their role and remit.
- MAWD has been used to develop Adaptations Agreements between local authorities and housing associations.
- MAWD is mentioned in a number of reports and guidance documents outside of England.

However, the review of MAWD also found that:

- In practice some housing associations are still referring to occupational therapy teams.
- Occupational therapists want to work in creative ways (beyond working with housing associations), but MAWD does not provide reassurance or guidance on how to do this.
- The process of providing (minor) adaptations without an occupational therapy assessment has not generally been broadened to apply across tenure.

Findings in relation to the common issues across the four UK nations about the process of providing adaptations included:

- There continue to be delays in the delivery of minor adaptations for people in private tenures.

- There continue to be delays in the delivery of major adaptations across tenure.

- Some housing associations are not providing minor adaptations without an occupational therapy assessment.

- Across the four UK nations, adaptations are defined by type (minor/major) and cost rather than being defined by the complexity of the individual's circumstances (i.e. related to their needs and home environment).

- There are varying levels of skills and competence among individuals signposting at first points of contact in housing, health, social care and the private sector.

- There continues to be a lack of information for individuals about adaptations: how to decide what they might need, when to consult an occupational therapist, what funding is available and who can carry out the work.

Findings in relation to the gaps stakeholders identified in the original publication included:

- MAWD does not provide sufficient guidance on the criteria for when and why an occupational therapist is or is not needed.

- The existing guidance is primarily focused on housing associations and their tenants.

- The existing guidance is paper-based; an online version is now required.

- The existing guidance is less applicable to Northern Ireland, Scotland and Wales than to England.

Findings in relation to the content and resources required in a new *Adaptations without delay* guide included:

- A framework for decision making that is based on the complexity of the 'case' in relation to adaptations.

- A reasoning framework for when an occupational therapist *is not* needed.

- In both cases (above), guidance about when an occupational therapy assessment is not required for recommending different types of adaptations.

- A definition of minor and major adaptations that is not based on cost.

- Updated examples of good practice in the delivery of adaptations.

- Recommended training/competencies, particularly for non-occupational therapists who may be able to recommend adaptations.

- A guide that is applicable across all four UK nations.

The discussion groups specifically identified the disproportionate use of specialist (i.e. occupational therapist) skills in relation to the assessment for and provision of adaptations as an issue that this new guide should address.

This review identified an ongoing need for practical guidance in relation to the assessment for and provision of adaptations more generally, beyond existing categorisations of 'minor' and 'major' adaptations, across all tenures. The review identified a need for this guide to provide a framework for decision making about adaptations based on the level and degree of *complexity* rather than more traditional minor/major adaptation and cost-based definitions.

About the authors

Rachel Russell PHd, MSc, BSc (Hons) Occupational Therapy

Rachel is an occupational therapist, lecturer and researcher based at the University of Salford. With 18 years' experience of working in adult health and social care, she has been directly involved in the assessment and delivery of home adaptations in several local authorities. Since 2011, her research has focused on the home adaptations process in the UK, particularly the role of occupational therapists in this process.

Marney Walker DipCOT, BA, MA

Marney Walker is an independent occupational therapist with 25 years' experience in housing and social care. She specialises in advising on the design of inclusive and accessible housing and adaptations. She has an MA in Design Research for Disability and has taught at master's level. She hosts a web page of resources on the Housing LIN Design Hub, is an Inclusive Design Assessor for the Civic Trust and a member of the Access Association.

Ian Copeman BSc, MSc

Ian leads the Housing LIN's programme of research and commercial consultancy. He has previously worked as a local authority commissioner of housing and care services, for housing associations and for voluntary sector organisations that support people with disabilities.

He has an extensive track record of undertaking research projects in housing and care in relation to older and disabled people. His recent projects with a high public profile include working in a consortium with Ipsos MORI on the Department of Work and Pensions and the Department of Communities and Local Government Supported Accommodation Review across England, Scotland and Wales. He is the author of the National Housing Federation's *Home from hospital* report and the Local Government Association's *Housing our ageing population* report.

He has previously been a trustee of a charity that provides housing advice and support for people with learning disabilities and their families.

Jeremy Porteus FRSA, Chief Executive, Housing LIN

Jeremy was formerly National Lead for Housing at the Department of Health responsible for the Extra Care Housing capital programme. After leaving the department, he founded the independent Housing LIN (Learning and Improvement Network), bringing together over 25,000 housing, health and social care practitioners in England, Wales and Scotland to identify and showcase innovative housing solutions for an ageing population.

The Housing LIN's free knowledge- and information-sharing activities, along with its consultancy business, provide market insight and intelligence on the latest funding, research, policy and practice to inspire better housing and care choices.

Jeremy is Inquiry Secretariat and author of the influential HAPP12, HAPPI3 and HAPPI4 reports for the All Party Parliamentary Group on Housing and Care for Older People. He also co-authored RIBA's 2018 publication: *Age-friendly housing: Future design for older people*.

https://www.housinglin.org.uk

Steering group members

Sue Adams OBE
Chief Executive, Care & Repair England

Paul Cooper
Professor Advisor – Practice, Royal College of Occupational Therapists

Ian Copeman
Principal Associate, Housing LIN

Jenny Davies
Occupational Therapist, Independent Practitioner

Welsh Representative, RCOTSS – Housing

Sarah Davies
Senior Policy and Practice Office, Chartered Institute of Housing

Joanna Gillies
Occupational Therapist

Scotland Representative, RCOTSS – Housing

Eve Parkinson
Head of Adult Services, Monmouthshire County Council

RCOT Welsh Board member

Jill Pritchard
Change Management Practitioner

Scotland Representative, RCOTSS – Housing

Dr Rachel Russell
Occupational Therapist, University of Salford

Julia Skelton
Director of Professional Operations, Royal College of Occupational Therapists

Paul Smith
Director, Foundations

Mary Stobie
Occupational Therapist

Northern Ireland Representative, RCOTSS – Housing

Marney Walker
Independent Occupational Therapist

Philippa Winstanley
Service Manager – Promoting Independent Living Services, Herefordshire Council

England Representative, RCOTSS – Housing.